Printed in the United States of America

First Printing, 2013

ISBN-13: 978-1482660593
ISBN-10: 1482660598

www.acheivingpeace.net
www.fitn40crew.com

All scriptures references are taken from the
THE HOLY BIBLE, NEW INTERNATIONAL
VERSION®, NIV® Copyright © 1973, 1978, 1984, 2011
by Biblica, Inc.™ Used by permission.
All rights reserved worldwide.

Concept and consulting provided by
Javaun Jackson
consultjavaun@gmail.com

Design and Artwork/Graphics by ChavonNachelle
www.chavonnachelle.com

WHAT PEOPLE ARE SAYING

"I think this is an awesome piece of work!"
-Jackie Washington
USA Olympian and Hall of Famer

"Yolanda is purposed to make the pain of the process pleasurable for its' designed purpose. She made a believer out of me!"
-Pastor Johnasen Pack
Bridge Builders International Church
Jordan Partnership

"Yolanda has poured her heart and soul into the pages of this fitness devotional. It is inspiring, thought-provoking and most importantly full of the Word of God. This devotional will bring change to the lives of the thousands who read its pages."
-Pastor Nero & Elect Lady Pia Foster
Covenant Worship Center

"I knew it was a matter of time. The mark of greatness is all over Yolanda and every day of this devotional. This is excellent, but there's still so much more to come…and I can't wait!"
-Kevin Williams
Life, Health, & Prosperity Coach

"I'm very proud of Yolanda and what she's bringing to the fitness industry. A fresh face, energy, and excitement! Great job!"
-Floyd Heard
USA Olympian

ACKNOWLEDGEMENTS

Iron Sharpens Iron Team
Javaun Jackson, Kevin Williams,
Chavon Riggins, and Bobbia Lawrence
Thank you for believing in me, being there for guidance,
and bringing my vision to life.
What an awesome team!

The Harper Comedy Show
What can I say other than there is nothing like family and
ours is very special and because of YOU,
I AM and YOU are my favorite!
Let's always look to the angels!

My Sister Circle
Thank you for the laughs, talks, and never ending support
and confidence that I could really do this!

Fit&40 Crew
There are too many names to mention, experiences to
recall, and laughs to remember. For every workout, prayer, or
kind word of support, "thank you" does not cover the level of
appreciation and gratitude.

TABLE OF CONTENTS

INTRODUCTION

Every area of my life changed in 2008. I left an abusive marriage of three years, a job of eight years, a church of 10 years, and a community of 12 years. Talk about transition!!! To find my way through all these shifts and changes was very difficult for me and my daughter, Ashanti. From depression to being diagnosed as an emotionally battered woman, the road has been long and interesting to say the least, but something happened one morning as I began preparing for my day. I sat down and began to reflect on an euphoric feeling that had tears streaming down my face. They were grateful tears. They were content tears. They were tears of peace…a peace that surpassed all understanding. It was then that I began to reflect over each area of my life and became appreciative that although it was not a perfect life, it was a very peaceful life. My time was spent living an active, balanced, and healthy lifestyle. *Active* as in doing things on a daily basis that brought me joy and happiness in the forms of exercising and helping others become more fit and active. *Healthy* as in emotionally, financially, spiritually, mentally and physically strong. I had an intimate relationship with God and a great network of people around me who reciprocated empowerment, motivation and encouragement. My bank account wasn't much, but I didn't have any unmet needs and my wants were few. *Balanced* as in giving enough to each area of my life so that no part was lacking or neglected.

Please journey with me over the next 31 days as I share the road to achieving peace. It is my prayer that this devotional will be a blessing to you and lead you to a pathway of experiencing the same peace that surpasses all understanding.

~DAY 1~

"Let us not become weary in doing good, for at the proper time we will reap a harvest if we do not give up." Galatians 6:9

Honestly, there are mornings I simply do not feel like going to the gym. I want to stay in my comfortable bed, hit snooze and be like so many others and simply sleep in. When I quickly think about my goals and how hard I've worked thus far, I get myself together and head out. Not only are these some of the best workouts, but it doesn't take me long to realize a thought provoking concept. I often wonder how much would actually get done if I based my actions on *how I felt!* I'm sure I would not move to the sound of an alarm at 4:15 a.m. and I'm also sure my overall life would be hectic, crazy and out of control. In order to live an active, healthy and balanced lifestyle, I can't base my actions on my feelings because they change daily, by the moment. Instead, I have to keep my eyes on the prize, focus on my goals and operate at my highest level of potential...even when I don't feel like it.

My Strong Tower,

Call to Action
The next time you have a moment of "I don't feel like it" change your mind and say, "I'm focused on my goal!"

Affirmation
"I will operate at my highest potential because my goals are important!"

~DAY 2~

"I have heard that the spirit of the gods is in you and that you have insight, intelligence and outstanding wisdom." Daniel 5:14

There is a misconception about women who lift weights. I hear from my female clients, "I would like to tone up, but I don't want to look like a bodybuilder or man!" I would be rich if I had a dollar for every time I hear, or read this statement. Our world is overflowing with a wealth of information and we must begin to seek out that information and remove the myths and misconceptions about health and fitness. We must remove, "I don't know!" from our vocabulary when the answers are a search engine away. If you want to know how many daily calories you need to lose weight, a workout routine for a beginner or even if you want to know how many licks it takes to get to the center of a lollipop, guess what…the answer is at the tip of your fingers and a search engine away.

Omnipotent God,

Call to Action
Research an exercise routine for a body part you'd like to improve.

Affirmation
"I possess an endless supply of knowledge for any project I assume."

~DAY 3~

"So God created man in His own image, in the image of God He created them; male and female he created them." Genesis 1:27

The point of going to the gym is to sweat and get healthy and in great shape right? Well, why not look stylish and fabulous while doing it, especially if we carefully choose our ensembles for other events and occasions like important meetings and Sunday worship services. What we decide to wear each day affects the way we think, the way we feel, the way we act and the way others react to us. Take a few minutes each night to plan and coordinate workout clothes just like preparing for other interactions with the outside world. Take pride in what you're wearing…even while you're in the gym sweating. Afterall, if we look good, we'll feel good too!

Jesus,

Call to Action
Purchase new workout gear including shoes.

Affirmation
"I will make my appearance important!"

~DAY 4~

"He replied, "Because you have so little faith. Truly I tell you, if you have faith as small as a mustard seed, you can say to this mountain, 'Move from here to there,' and it will move. Nothing will be impossible for you." Matthew 17:20

There's something about this "faith" thing that could be beneficial along this journey. We can apply faith to our discipline that is required to stay committed to an active lifestyle. To truly believe in a goal that we have yet to accomplish, but continue day to day working towards can sometimes be discouraging. A mustard seed of faith planted along with commitment and determination is imperative in pursuing this journey to a successful end. Speak life and call things into existence then wait for the full manifestation. It works in other areas of our lives so when we limit ourselves, we limit God and that is a disservice to everyone.

Faithful Father,

Call to Action
Believe God for something you desire and do not waiver in your faith, then watch God move.

Affirmation
"I believe in me!"

~DAY 5~

"…but those who hope in the LORD will renew their strength.
They will soar on wings like eagles; they will run and not grow weary, they will
walk and not be faint." Isaiah 40:31

When initially faced with the challenges of life, it's not time to question our own ability, but having faith in God that we have the strength to overcome every circumstance. Because of this power within us, we should never settle for anything less than the very best God has to offer…inside or outside the gym. This knowledge will allow for an extra set, greater intensity or even more endurance. At first attempt, it might seem difficult, but if we tap into that inner strength we will no longer settle for mediocrity…inside or outside the gym. Today would be a great day to take the usual mundane workout to another level. Are you ready?

Powerful God,

Call to Action
Find a way to challenge yourself inside or outside the gym.

Affirmation
"I am better and stronger!"

~DAY 6~

"Forgetting what is behind and straining toward what is ahead, I press on toward the goal to win the prize for which God has called me heavenward in Christ Jesus." Philippians 3:13-14

Even in life, there are times when we feel as if we are stuck and simply going through the motions. In fitness, it's called, "hitting a plateau." The only way to press past the plateau is to press harder, dig deeper, lift heavier and eat cleaner. You don't just stay there because it's comfortable because when you want more, you take the necessary steps to do more. Step out of the comfort zone and try something different and more challenging. Whether it's a different strength training routine, group class or boot camp; whatever you decide allow it to expand past the comfort zone and push you beyond that comfortable place. After all, we are champions!

My Redeemer,

Call to Action
Do something you would never do.

Affirmation
"I will step outside my comfort zone!"

~DAY 7~

"Two are better than one, because they have a good return for their labor. If either of them falls down, one can help the other up. But pity anyone who falls and has no one to help them up." Ecclesiastes 4:9-10

Who holds you accountable? Who tells you when you're right or wrong? Who do you have in your life that won't allow you the opportunity to settle or not give your very best? Accountability partners/mentors are imperative to your success. When I'm tired and my body says, "ENOUGH," my workout buddy is there at the right time to say, "You got this!" And just as soon as I hear those words, what action follows? I take a deep breath, give it all that I have left and respond with, "I sure do!" Now is not the time to surround ourselves with, "YES" people, but with those who will push us when we want to give up.

Most Excellent One,

Call to Action
Tell your accountability partner/workout buddy/mentor
"Thank you for the push!"

Affirmation
"I will push and be pushed to excellence!"

~DAY 8~

"Consider it pure joy, my brothers and sisters, whenever you face trials of many kinds, because you know that the testing of your faith produces perseverance. Let perseverance finish its work so that you may be mature and complete, not lacking anything." James 1:2-4

Oftentimes, goals are not met because we overwhelm ourselves with attempting too much change at one time and the absence of "stick-to-it-tiveness." We simply give up when we are confronted with a challenge, fall short or even have a bad day. We are too quick to throw in the towel and wave the white flag at the very sight of adversity. Where is the "ain't no stopping me now!" attitude? What happened to, "Whatever it takes to get the job done!?" Do not stamp failure on the weight loss journey or healthy lifestyle until every effort has been made to be successful- not 50% or 75%, but 100% effort in every area: nutrition, sleep and exercise.

My Refuge,

Call to Action
Recall the feeling when you overcame a difficult challenge.

Affirmation
"I believe my body is strong and body willing!"

~DAY 9~

"I have fought a good fight, I have finished the race, I have kept the faith." 2 Timothy 4:7

I was in the gym one morning finishing up a grueling leg workout that consisted of carrying a 70lb bar while doing walking lunges around the perimeter of the gym, when an older gentleman said, "Young lady, I don't know how you do it! I get tired just watching you!" I smiled and responded, "Thank you," and as I stepped forward, I questioned myself as I felt my shoulders and legs reaching fatigue. It's one lunge at a time. Yes, one foot in front of the other. It hurt and burned, but I continued with one step at a time. I wiped my sweat, took a deep breath and answered the question with, "I can do all things through Christ. I can do all things through Christ. I can do all things through Christ!" That's how I do it! One step at a time, knowing that I can do all things through HIM!

Jehovah Rohi,

Call to Action
Go farther than yesterday.

Affirmation
"I have everything I need to exceed any obstacle I face!"

~DAY 10~

*"Trust in the LORD with all your heart and lean not
on your own understanding; in all your ways submit to him,
and he will make your paths straight." Proverbs 3:5-6*

I introduced a new piece of equipment to my crew which was a gently used fire hose and before even attempting the drill, a crew member stated, "I can't do that. It's too heavy!" I walked towards her and made direct eye contact and said, "So you're going to give up before you even try?" She looked at the hose then back at me. My stare was more intense and she knew I meant business when I said, "Now get over there, dig deep and give me everything you've got!" She walked toward the hose, adjusted her hands and I shouted, "GO!" as I hit the stopwatch. The intensity in her face was priceless as she soon caught onto the rhythm as the seconds ticked by! I shouted "STOP!" but she kept going! The crew and I encouraged her to continue while she let out loud grunts and moans. She then dropped the hose and a huge smile came across her face. She turned in our direction and said, "WOW! That felt so good. I did it Yolanda. I did it!"

Precious Lord,

Call to Action
Experience something new.

Affirmation
"I am more powerful than I believe!"

~DAY 11~

"But he was pierced for our transgressions, he was crushed for our iniquities; the punishment that brought us peace was upon him, and by his wounds we are healed." Isaiah 53:5

What is your reality? Mine is cancer that runs rampant through my maternal bloodline. My mother is a two-time colon cancer survivor, my maternal grandmother died of a cancerous brain tumor, and my maternal grandfather passed away due to colon cancer. According to statistics, I have a very high probability of getting diagnosed with the horrid disease. The blood of Jesus covers me and I can break this curse. I made a promise to myself that as long as I have strength in my body, I will do everything within my power to avoid sitting across from a doctor and hearing those words, "This could have been avoided with proper diet and exercise!"

My Shield,

Call to Action
Pray over any generational medical curse that's in your bloodline.

Affirmation
"I have the ability to change my life!"

~DAY 12~

"The one who plants and the one who waters have one purpose, and they will each be rewarded according to their own labor."
1 Corinthians 3:8

It's time out for making excuses of why we can't live our best life. It's no longer the fault of past generations, our schedules or anything else…sometimes it's simply US holding ourselves back from reaching our goals and living on purpose. We tell ourselves we can't and then find reasons or excuses to support the seed of doubt. We just have to change our mindset…simple as that. Instead of thinking of ways it can't be done or why we can't be successful, attach the feeling of completion and victory to it and begin to explore ways it CAN be done. Like the famous shoe slogan states, "Just do it!"

Prince of Peace,

Call to Action
Offer an option when faced with the next challenge.

Affirmation
"I will focus on the end result and reward!"

~DAY 13~

"Whether you turn to the right or to the left, your ears will hear a voice behind you, saying, 'This is the way; walk in it.'" Isaiah 30:21

I remember watching cartoons as a child. When the character was faced with a decision, a puff of smoke with a "devil" would appear on one shoulder then another puff of smoke with an "angel" would appear on the opposite shoulder. The character was in a state of confusion as he first listened to the little devil on the left, and then quickly turned and listened to the little angel on the right. More often than not, the character went with the wrong decision, which left him in more trouble than expected. The same issue would appear again later but this time, he pushed the little devil off of his shoulder and went with the better, more wise decision of the angel. This journey is not easy and we must be careful who we allow to "speak to us." Who are we listening to and where are they guiding us? We are influenced by outside events and people, but what about listening to our own heart and that still and quiet voice that leads us down the right path saying, "This is the way; walk in it!"

My Well of Living Water,

Call to Action
Recognize the naysayers.

Affirmation
"I will be quiet and listen for direction!"

~DAY 14~

"As iron sharpens iron, so one person sharpens another."
Proverbs 27:17

A habit is an acquired behavior pattern regularly followed until it has become almost involuntary. We have made "lazy" a habit by being inactive and sedentary. Gone are the days of outside activities. Technology has created higher statistics of obesity and diseases and the conditions associated with them. As we make it a habit to exercise and do things that will continue to challenge our bodies, it is imperative that we surround ourselves with other like-minded people who are doing things we enjoy or would like to try. These are the people who will remind us of our goals, workouts, successes, challenges and new ideas. These are the people who will hold us accountable and not accept any excuses. Just as iron sharpens iron, so does lazy sharpen lazy.

My Rock,

Call to Action
Encourage those around you to get active.

Affirmation
"I will be accountable to someone!"

~DAY 15~

"And let us consider how to spur one another on toward love and good deeds." Hebrews 10:24

While sitting in the steam room one morning, a lady sat next to me and said, "I didn't feel like coming to the gym this morning, but I did and I saw you working out hard. You motivated me to step up my game, and I got it together and put forth a better effort!" She didn't know I was 45 minutes late and almost decided against a morning session. It was in that moment that I realized that people are watching us and drawing from our energy and spirit even when we don't realize it. Usually people just watch without saying anything, but I was fortunate she actually shared this with me because it was refreshing to hear. It gave me a little extra encouragement as well. So smile, hold your head up and radiate a positive spirit because somebody is watching.

Everlasting Father,

Call to Action
Say something encouraging to someone.

Affirmation
"I will be encouraged as I encourage others!"

~DAY 16~

"The plans of the diligent lead surely to profit as surely as haste leads to poverty."
Proverbs 21:5

When we plan a vacation, we research the location, method of travel, hotel accommodations and the many other details that will ensure an awesome time is had by all. Can you imagine if we carefully planned other areas of our lives in the same manner, specifically our exercise programs? Think about a time when we finally made up our mind to do something and how good we felt once it was accomplished. Whether big or small, we didn't let anyone or anything deter us from pursuing it with full force. Can you imagine what kind of life we would have if we applied this same tenacity and mindset in reaching our goals?

Jehovah Adonai,

Call to Action
Pay attention to the details of day to day life.

Affirmation
"I am committed to healthy behaviors!"

~DAY 17~

"Then the Lord replied: "Write down the revelation and write it plain on tablets so that a herald may run who reads it." Habakkuk 2:2

The S.M.A.R.T. (Specific, Measureable, Attainable, Realistic, Time-based) goal-setting method, in the 7 Habits of Highly Effective People by Stephen Covey, is a very effective planning tool. It allows seeing the big picture while breaking it down into smaller steps to achieve success along the way. So the question, "How do you eat an elephant?" is no longer an overwhelming task when this method is applied while we reach the conclusion, "One bite at a time." Oftentimes, our goals can seem overwhelming, unrealistic, or even out of reach. This is a sure setup for failure, but when we concentrate on one bite at a time and celebrate the small successes along the way, we can sit back in satisfaction knowing that we followed the path and met the desired outcome.

Jehovah,

Call to Action
Create a S.M.A.R.T. goal on page 38.

Affirmation
"I have everything necessary to succeed!"

~DAY 18~

God is our refuge and strength, an ever-present help in trouble.
Psalm 46:1

There are two to three fitness magazines that I love to read regularly because they each offer something different. I enjoy reading the articles, healthy recipes, trying new workouts and even imagining myself as one of the female models. The magazines not only keep me motivated but also serve as a reminder that it's truly a lifestyle. When people make good and healthy choices, they live longer, feel better, generally more well-balanced and happier people. Think about your own life over the past 30 days and how it has changed. It may be simple things such as sleeping better, increased energy and greater confidence. I keep my magazines all over my house as a constant reminder of why it's so important to find things that bring me joy…like working out!

Heavenly Father,

Call to Action
Visit a fitness website for helpful articles or recipes.

Affirmation
"I am fit, healthy and attractive!"

~DAY 19~

"But I tell you that everyone will have to give account on the day of judgement for every empty word they have spoken." Matthew 12:36

"If you don't have anything good to say, then don't say anything at all!" Many can count the numerous times this echoed throughout our childhood. Usually it was referring to someone else, but what about the nasty and unkind things we say to ourselves? We complain about our thighs, core and flabby chicken wing arms. Why not take a few minutes to admire them? Let's not complain about the things we allow and instead give ourselves permission to change, be happy and successful with our bodies and in life. What are you saying to yourself that is perpetuating the belief that you can't or won't reach your goals? Remember, "If you don't have anything good to say…"

My Shepherd,

Call to Action
Put a silver coin in a jar each time negative self-talk occurs.

Affirmation
"I will speak words that build."

~DAY 20~

"Do you not know that your bodies are temples of the Holy Spirit, who is in you, whom you have received from God? You are not your own; you were bought at a price. Therefore honor God with your bodies." 1 Corinthians 6:19-20

Imagine we left our house to a friend while we were away and it was a mess by the time we returned. From the front door to the back door, it was cluttered with newspapers, dirty dishes in the sink and an overall dump. Can you imagine the conversation? "What happened to my house? I trusted you would take care of it! I trusted you to keep it clean and in good shape!" Now, imagine a conversation God is having with us about the way we have treated our bodies: His temple. We must ensure we are supplying our bodies with nutritious food that is energy to our temples instead of feeding it with food containing poisonous toxic substances and by-products. When we are full of energy, we are more mentally alert and physically strong to carry out our daily assignments.

Lifter of my head,

Call to Action
Give your internal house a good cleaning.

Affirmation
"I will use food for energy and not pleasure!"

~DAY 21~

"I praise you because I am fearfully and wonderfully made; your works are wonderful, I know that full well." Psalm 139:14

We are all very different and society has played a huge role in how we view others and ourselves. We have different mindsets, interpret things differently, have different emotions and experiences. From flawless skin to six pack abs, we often have an image of an idealistic lifestyle or body type. When we compare ourselves to others in any manner, we discount our own natural beauty and uniqueness. This can also take away the right to be in love with who we are and everything that makes us so special...even our bodies. There is only one YOU and in all your uniqueness, appreciate that you are fearfully and wonderfully made. So smile at the image in the mirror and say, "I'm going to adore these hips and thighs because they're mine, all mine!"

Alpha & Omega,

Call to Action
Write a positive statement about the body
part you least admire.

Affirmation
"I am simply amazing and awesome!"

"For we must all appear before the judgement seat of Christ, that each one may receive what is due him for the things done while in the body, whether good or bad." 2 Corinthians 5:10

There is an area in each of our lives that we wish were a little different. There are issues that have been ignored that disappear briefly but seem to reappear at any given moment. We all have that "something." MY something might not be YOURS, so does that make one greater than the next? NO, it just confirms we are all human and we all have SOMETHING! When we judge ourselves or others, we put pressure on day to day living by setting an unfair standard or stereotype. Instead of accepting how things are, we focus on how things should be overlooking the fact that things are happening according to God's schedule and not ours. Life could be much more simple if we strive to judge less, forgive more, monitor our thoughts and look for the positive, in ourselves and others.

My Dwelling Place,

Call to Action
Forgive those whom you've judged.

Affirmation
"I will not judge myself or others!"

~DAY 23~

"Remember this: Whoever sows sparingly will also reap sparingly, and whoever sows generously will also reap generously." 2 Corinthians 9:6

Although our economy has dictated different financial decisions for many people, it is very evident that people will always spend their money where they see fit. Whether it's shopping, dining out or traveling, people will always find a means to an end when there is an interest. Unfortunately, this does not always apply to our health. The first quarter of each year there is always an increase in gym memberships across the country, but what about investing that same money and determination throughout the year by hiring a personal trainer or participating in a local boot camp? It's an awesome feeling to look good on the outside, but even more rewarding when the inside matches.

Jehovah Jireh,

Call to Action
Hire a fitness or health professional.

Affirmation
"I'm worth it and owe it to myself!"

"For I know the plans I have for you, declares the Lord, 'plans to prosper you and not to harm you, plans to give you hope and a future.'" Jeremiah 29:11

I read in a fitness magazine, "When you improve your self-esteem, you'll take better care of yourself." I thought about the many underlying issues that prevent us from being successful in any area of our lives. Whether it's the inner voice of childhood being told "we couldn't", life experiences, the fear of failure or the fear of success, there is something that acts as a barrier for each of us. Another relative reading I came across stated, "You cannot be successful with unforgiveness in your heart!" Wow! We can't move forward and be successful when we carry the guilt, condemnation, hurt, and unresolved issues of our past. Let's recognize the barrier and get over it. It happened and we are all the better and stronger because it did.

Almighty Savior,

Call to Action
Let it go!

Affirmation
"I am open to forgive myself and others!"

~DAY 25~

"Therefore, if anyone is in Christ, the new creation has come: The old has gone, the new is here!" 2 Corinthians 5:17

Once I reached my weight loss goal, I found my morning routine *"frustrating!"* I tried on item after item of clothing that hung over my frame like a draped cloth. Even when I looked at the size, for some reason, I still slid them on like the number didn't matter…but it did. One day while training a client and discussing HER recent weight loss progress, she mentioned she could no longer wear any of her clothes and was the exact size that now crowded my closet. I told her, "I will have something for you the next time I see you!" She had no idea I was about to remove this same frustration from her morning routine. When I got home, I immediately started gathering all the items from my closet that I could no longer wear. I guess deep down inside, I was having a hard time accepting my new body and letting the old things go, but my frustration was now someone else's blessing.

Almighty God,

Call to Action
Take gently used clothing to a local shelter.

Affirmation
"I have things that will be a blessing to others."

~DAY 26~

"Do not conform to the pattern of this world, but be transformed by the renewing of your mind. Then you will be able to test and approve what God's will is-his good, pleasing and perfect will." Romans 12:2

Usually, women are conditioned as nurturers and accustomed to taking care of everyone and everything. It was selfish of us if we didn't…or so we were taught. However, if we can schedule the kids' practices, medical appointments, family errands, household necessities, and quality time with our significant others surely we can schedule some time for just US…and do with that time whatever WE please. While •we might not always have time for a walk or uninterrupted bubble bath, taking a few minutes a day is essential to maintaining our sanity and the wellness of those around us. It's our responsibility to ensure the every area is taken care of, but above all, we owe it to ourselves to take a breather as needed. It's all about living a healthy, active and BALANCED lifestyle. The lack of balance in our lives may be the reasons so many are frustrated, depressed, resentful and fatigued!

Holy One,

Call to Action
Be still and quiet.

Affirmation
"I will schedule consistent time for myself!"

~DAY 27~

"For God is not a God of disorder but of peace-as in all the congregations of the Lord's people." 1 Corinthians 14:33

For many, life is about happiness and fulfillment. These are the things that make us feel as if our time has been well spent; a result, they motivate many of the decisions we make. To achieve happiness and fulfillment, you must somehow benefit mentally and/or physically from your actions. Your loved ones will see that you are serious about this lifestyle change and respect the time you request. Let it be about you and make yourself proud! It's not called "selfish" when you're working on being balanced.

Peaceful God,

Call to Action
Create a quiet space to call your own.

Affirmation
"I am successful at reaching my goals!"

~DAY 28~

"Each one should test his own actions. Then he can take pride himself, without comparing himself to somebody else…" Galatians 6:4

Our goal is to be the healthiest and strongest we can possibly be at whatever age or stage we are in life. Even though we have our families and friends who are important to us and we want to share a long and happy life with, at the end of the day, we are our own responsibility and competition. From a balanced perspective, it is an opportunity to discern differences in order to focus on uniqueness and workout partners and role models are a great help. When used as a resource, the goal is to find areas to strengthen and not weaken. Healthy competition says, "Let's push each other so we can all become better!" while unhealthy competition says, "I'm better than you!" Remember, you are your own competition!

My Strength,

Call to Action
Find a healthy workout partner or mentor.

Affirmation
"I am my own competition!"

~DAY 29~

"...because you know that the Lord will reward each one for whatever good they do, whether they are slave or free." Ephesians 6:8

We are an individualist society consumed with the: "me, my four, and no more" syndrome. At what point are we going to see that someone else might be in need? When are we going to look around and say, "I've come a very long way, I've learned a few things about fitness, exercise and nutrition and let me see if I can help someone else along the way." There's someone who sees something in us they wish they could have as part of their journey! When are we going to reach out a hand and say, "She's not heavy, she's my sister!" We all need people who have traveled the road before us, and as we open ourselves up to give or help another, we make room to be filled again and again.

My Advocate,

Call to Action
Help someone in need.

Affirmation
"I have a lot to offer others in need!"

~DAY 30~

"...then make my joy complete by being like-minded, having the same love, being one in spirit and of one mind." Philippians 2:2

While playing with magnets, I realized that one side quickly attracted and connected with the other, but when I turned one over, there seemed to be a force that would not allow them to connect. When the two sides connected, there was something in common that brought them together, while the opposing sides had nothing in common. Our lives are very much like these magnets: we attract what is inside of us. If happiness, abundance, wealth, prosperity, health, and peace are within us, that is what will come to us. If none of these things are in our lives, we are left with lack, emptiness, misery and negativity, which are all opposing elements to living an active, healthy and balanced lifestyle.

Everlasting Father,

Call to Action
Surround yourself with positive & prospering people.

Affirmation
"My circle of friends is a direct reflection of who I am!"

~DAY 31~

"In peace I will both lie down and sleep; for you alone, O Lord, make me dwell in safety." Psalm 4:8

What feeling do you get when you walk into your bedroom? How would you describe it to someone? Is it a peaceful environment that invites rest and sleep or is it filled with clothes and other clutter? We should spend approximately 6-8 hours every night in bed resting or asleep, and it should be comfortable from the mattress, sheets and pillows to the proper lighting. Our bedroom should be a tranquil environment that will allow our bodies to slow down and rest as we slip into a state of peaceful sleep. When we wake up in the morning, we should be energized and ready to take on the world, not sluggish hitting the alarm over and over. This time is very important as it also allows our muscles to repair themselves. We need both rest and sleep in order to operate at our highest potential.

Jehovah Shalom,

Call to Action
Invest in new bedding or décor.

Affirmation
"My bedroom is a place of peace and comfort!"

APPENDIX

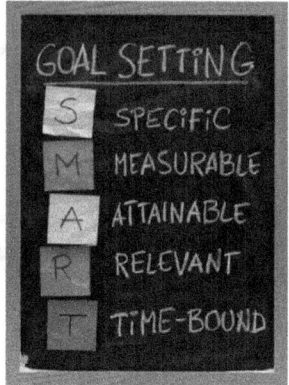

Specific: What are you going to do?
Measurable: How will you reach your goal?
Attainable: Is it important?
Relevant: Is it realistic?
Time-bound: When will you complete it?

Example: "I want to lose 20lbs in 90 days. I will perform 30 minutes of cardio and 30 minutes of strength training per day, 5 days a week, and I will only eat starchy carbohydrates 3 times per week.

Practice writing a goal using this method.

_____
_____
_____
_____
_____
_____
_____
_____
_____
_____
_____
_____

ABOUT THE AUTHOR

Born in Fort Worth, Texas, Yolanda has always been athletic, even dating back to field day in elementary school. Throughout her school aged years, she actively participated in organized athletics from volleyball, to basketball, to track and field, her favorite. Yolanda's talent and passion led to her being recognized as a top female athlete in the DFW area. As a result, she received a full athletic scholarship to the University of Houston where she trained with Olympic greats Carl Lewis, LeRoy Burrell, and Floyd Heard, just to name a few. Her athletic career also allowed her the opportunity to compete against track and field's elite women athletes Jackie Joyner-Kersee, Gail Devers, and many others.

Yolanda has established herself as a writer and motivational speaker and has been featured in local printed publications. Her enjoyment for uplifting and encouraging others through life has provided countless opportunities for other motivational speaking events in the DFW area. Her extensive background includes: women's Bible study teacher, youth track coach, athletic performance and personal training and AFAA certified group fitness instructor.

She lives in Grand Prairie, Texas and is the proud mother of Ashanti and doting grandmother of Bentley.

Please visit website at **www.fitn40crew.com** for details on her current outdoor fitness boot camp sessions.

www.ingramcontent.com/pod-product-compliance
Lightning Source LLC
Chambersburg PA
CBHW070512290526
45790CB00003B/1198